COOK BOOK MUG RECIPE ON MICROWAVE FOR COLLEGE STUDENTS AND WORKING CLASS

30 tested and trusted meal guides for quick and easy mug recipe for college students and working class people

AUTHOR ONI JOSEPH OLUSESAN

Table of Contents

INTRODUCTION

Microwave recipe cookbooks offer invaluable benefits for households and college students alike. Firstly, they provide convenience by offering quick and easy meal options suitable for busy schedules, making meal preparation hassle-free. Secondly, microwave recipes.

Promote healthier eating habits as they often emphasize fresh ingredients and efficient cooking methods, reducing the reliance on processed foods. Additionally, these cookbooks cater to diverse dietary preferences, including vegetarian, vegan, and gluten-free options, ensuring inclusivity and adaptability. For college students, microwave recipes are budget-friendly, requiring minimal ingredients and kitchen equipment, making them ideal for dorm room cooking. They also foster independence and culinary skills development among students, empowering them to prepare nutritious meals with limited resources. Overall, microwave recipe cookbooks offer practical solutions for individuals seeking efficiency, health consciousness, and culinary exploration in their everyday cooking routines.

CHPTER 1

Microwave scrambled eggs

Microwave scrambled eggs offer a convenient and speedy breakfast choice that can be made within minutes using a microwave-safe bowl or mug. Below is a comprehensive guide detailing the process of making microwave scrambled eggs.

- **Ingredients:**

2 eggs

2 tablespoons of milk or water Salt and pepper (to taste) Optional: shredded cheese, diced vegetables, cooked bacon or ham, herbs, etc.

- **Instructions:**
- Begin by cracking two eggs into a microwave-safe bowl or mug. Ensure that the container is of sufficient size to prevent the eggs from overflowing while cooking.

- Use a fork or whisk to thoroughly beat three eggs until the yolks and whites are well blended. This will result in a uniform texture for your scrambled eggs.

- Pour 2 tablespoons of milk or water into the beaten eggs. This addition will contribute to the fluffiness of the eggs and prevent them from becoming rubbery when cooked in the microwave.

- Season the egg mixture with salt and pepper according to your taste preferences. Additionally, you may incorporate any desired seasonings or herbs at this stage, such as chopped chives or parsley.

- If desired, add any additional fillings, such as shredded cheese, diced vegetables, or cooked bacon or ham, to the egg mixture. Stir them in thoroughly.

- Place the bowl or mug in the microwave and cook on high power for 30 seconds.

- After 30 seconds, remove the bowl or mug from the microwave and stir the eggs using a fork or spoon. This step helps ensure even cooking and prevents the edges from becoming overcooked.

- Return the bowl or mug to the microwave and continue cooking in intervals of 20 to 30 seconds, stirring after each interval. Stop when the eggs are almost set but still slightly runny.

- To determine if the eggs are cooked through, gently press a fork into the center of the scrambled eggs. If no liquid egg remains and the eggs are firm yet moist, they are done.

- Allow the scrambled eggs to rest for a minute or two before serving. This resting period will complete the cooking process, and the eggs will firm up slightly. Serve hot with toast, tortillas, or your preferred breakfast accompaniments.

- Microwave-scrambled eggs provide versatility as they allow for customization.

CHAPTER 2

Microwave Mug Omelets

Microwave mug omelets are a quick and easy breakfast option that can be prepared in just a few minutes using common ingredients and a microwave-safe mug. Here's a detailed explanation of how to prepare microwave mug omelets:

- **Ingredients:**
- 2 large eggs
- 2 tablespoons of milk
- Salt and pepper to taste
- Fillings of your choice (such as diced vegetables, cooked meats, shredded cheese, or herbs)
- **Instructions:**

1. **Prepare Your Mug**: Choose a microwave-safe mug that is large enough to hold the ingredients without overflowing. You can lightly grease the inside of the mug with cooking spray or butter to prevent sticking.
2. **Beat Eggs**: Crack two large eggs into the mug. Use a fork or small whisk to beat the eggs until they are well combined and slightly frothy.

3. **Add Milk and Seasonings**: Pour in 2 tablespoons of milk into the mug with the beaten eggs. Season with a pinch of salt and pepper, to taste. Whisk again briefly to incorporate the milk and seasonings into the eggs.

4. **Add Fillings**: Now it's time to add your desired fillings to the mug. This could include diced vegetables like bell peppers, onions, tomatoes, spinach, cooked meats like ham or bacon, and shredded cheese. You can customize the omelet with whatever ingredients you have on hand or prefer.

5. **Mix Fillings**: Use a fork or spoon to gently stir the fillings into the egg mixture, distributing them evenly throughout the mug.

6. **Microwave**: Place the mug in the microwave and cook on high power for about 1 to 2 minutes. Cooking time may vary depending on the wattage of your microwave, so keep an eye on the omelet as it cooks.

7. **Check for doneness**: After the initial cooking time, carefully remove the mug from the microwave and check the omelet's doneness. The edges should be set, and the center should be slightly firm. If it's still runny, return the mug to the microwave and cook in 30-second intervals until the omelet is fully cooked.

8. **Serve**: Once the omelet is cooked to your liking, carefully remove the mug from the microwave. Use a fork to loosen the edges of the omelet from the mug, and then gently slide it out onto a plate. Garnish with additional toppings, like fresh herbs or salsa, if desired.

9. **Enjoy**: Your microwave mug omelet is now ready to enjoy! Serve it hot and fresh for a quick and satisfying breakfast on the go.

- **Tips:**

1. Be sure to use a microwave-safe mug to avoid any risk of breakage or damage.
2. Customize your omelet with your favorite fillings for a personalized breakfast experience.

- Adjust the cooking time based on your microwave's wattage and the desired doneness of the omelet.
- Handle the mug carefully, as it will be hot after microwaving.
- Feel free to experiment with different herbs, spices, and sauces to add flavor to your omelet.
- Is this conversation helpful so far?

CHAPTER 3

Microwave-baked potato

- ○ **Ingredients**: potato, olive oil, salt

Method: Scrub the potato, poke holes, and rub with oil and salt. Microwave for 5–7 minutes, flipping halfway, until tender. ingredients:

Potato: Choose medium- to large-sized potatoes, such as russet or Yukon gold, depending on your preference.

Olive oil: Use a small amount of olive oil to rub over the potato skin. This helps to create a crispy exterior.

Salt: Sprinkle salt over the oiled potato for seasoning.

Method:

1. Scrub the potato: Thoroughly wash the potato under running water to remove any dirt or debris. Use a vegetable brush to scrub the skin clean.

2. Poke holes: Using a fork, poke several holes all around the potato. This allows steam to escape while the potato cooks, preventing it from bursting.

3. Rub with oil and salt: Drizzle a small amount of olive oil over the potato, then use your hands to rub it evenly over the skin. Sprinkle salt over the oiled potato, ensuring it's evenly coated.

4. Microwave: Place the prepared potato on a microwave-safe plate or dish. Microwave on high for 5-7 minutes, depending on the size of the potato and the power of your microwave. Remember to flip the potato halfway through the cooking time to ensure even cooking.

5. Check for doneness: After the initial cooking time, carefully remove the potato from the microwave and check for doneness. The potato should be tender when pierced with a fork or knife. If it's still firm in the center, continue microwaving in 1-minute increments until it's cooked to your liking.

6. Serve: Once the potato is cooked through, carefully remove it from the microwave. Allow it to cool for a few minutes before handling, as it will be hot. Serve the microwave baked potato with your favorite

toppings, such as butter, sour cream, cheese, chives or bacon bits.

Microwave baked potatoes are a convenient option for busy weeknights or when you're craving a quick and satisfying side dish. Experiment with different! seasonings and toppings to customize your potato to suit your taste preferences. Enjoy

CHAPTER 4

Microwave-steamed vegetables

- o **Ingredients:** assorted vegetables, water, salt
2. **Method:** Place vegetables in a microwave-safe dish with water and salt. Cover and microwave for 3-5 minutes until tender. Method:

1. Prepare the vegetables: Wash the vegetables thoroughly under running water to remove any dirt or debris. If using fresh vegetables, trim them and cut them into bite-sized pieces for even cooking. If using frozen vegetables, there's no need to thaw them before microwaving.

2. Place vegetables in a microwave-safe dish. Transfer the prepared vegetables to a microwave-safe dish. Make sure the dish is large enough to hold all the vegetables in a single layer, allowing them to cook evenly.

3. Add water and salt: Pour enough water into the dish to cover the bottom with a thin layer. The amount of water will depend on the quantity of vegetables you're cooking and the size of your dish. Sprinkle salt over

the vegetables for seasoning, if desired. The salt is optional but can enhance the flavor of the vegetables.

4. Cover the dish: Use a microwave-safe cover or microwave-safe plastic wrap to cover the dish. This helps to trap steam inside, which will cook the vegetables more quickly and evenly.

5. Microwave: Place the covered dish of vegetables in the microwave and cook on high power for 3-5 minutes. The exact cooking time will depend on the type and quantity of vegetables you're using, as well as the power of your microwave. Start with 3 minutes, then check for doneness. If the vegetables are still too firm, continue microwaving in 1-minute increments until they reach your desired level of tenderness.

6. Check for doneness: Carefully remove the dish from the microwave and uncover it. Use a fork or knife to pierce the vegetables and check for tenderness. They should be fork-tender but not mushy.

7. Serve: Once the vegetables are cooked to your liking, remove them from the microwave and serve immediately. You can enjoy them as a side dish, add them to salads, stir-fries, or pasta dishes, or use them as a topping for baked potatoes or grains.

Microwaving assorted vegetables is a quick and convenient way to prepare a nutritious side dish or add vegetables to your meals. Experiment with different vegetable combinations and seasonings to create delicious and healthy dishes. Enjoy!

CHAPTER 5

Microwave Macaroni and Cheese

- o **Ingredients:** macaroni, water, milk, cheese, salt, and pepper
- o **Method**: Combine macaroni and water in a microwave-safe bowl. Microwave in 2-minute intervals, stirring until cooked. Stir in milk, cheese, salt, and pepper. Certainly! Here's a more detailed explanation of how to make macaroni and cheese in the microwave:

2. **Ingredients:**

3. Macaroni: Use your preferred type of macaroni pasta, such as elbow macaroni or small shells.

4. Water: You'll need water to cook the macaroni.

5. Milk: Milk adds creaminess to the cheese sauce.

6. Cheese: Choose your favorite cheese or combination of cheeses for the sauce. Cheddar, mozzarella, or blends of cheeses work well.

7. Salt and pepper: These seasonings add flavor to the dish.

8. **Method:**

1. Combine macaroni and water: In a microwave-safe bowl, add the macaroni and enough water to cover the pasta completely. The ratio of water to pasta should be about 2:1. Stir to ensure the macaroni is submerged in the water.

2. Microwave in 2-minute intervals: Place the bowl of macaroni and water in the microwave and cook on high power in 2-minute intervals. After each interval, remove the bowl from the microwave and stir the macaroni. Continue microwaving and stirring until the macaroni is cooked to your desired level of tenderness. This typically takes about 6–8 minutes, depending on the power of your microwave and the type of pasta used.

3. Stir in the milk, cheese, salt, and pepper. Once the macaroni is cooked, carefully remove the bowl from the microwave. Stir in the milk and shredded cheese until the cheese is melted and forms a creamy sauce. Add salt and pepper to taste, adjusting the seasoning as needed.

4. Microwave to heat through (optional): If the cheese sauce needs to be heated further or if you prefer a hotter dish, you can microwave the macaroni and

cheese for an additional 1-2 minutes on high power, stirring halfway through.

5. Serve: Once the macaroni and cheese are heated through and the sauce is creamy and smooth, it's ready to serve. Enjoy it as a comforting and satisfying meal or side dish.

Making macaroni and cheese in the microwave is a quick and convenient way to satisfy your craving for this classic comfort food. Customize the recipe by adding cooked bacon, diced vegetables, or breadcrumbs for extra flavor and texture. Experiment with different cheeses to create your own unique macaroni-and-cheese masterpiece. Top of Form

CHATER 6

Microwave Mug Brownie

- **Ingredients:** flour, sugar, cocoa powder, oil, and water
- **Method:** Mix dry ingredients in a mug, add oil and water. Microwave for 1-2 minutes until set.

Here's a more detailed explanation of how to make a microwave mug brownie:

- **Ingredients:**
- Flour: All-purpose flour is commonly used for brownie recipes.
- Sugar: Granulated sugar adds sweetness to the brownie.
- Cocoa powder: Unsweetened cocoa powder provides the chocolate flavor.
- Oil: Vegetable oil or melted butter adds moisture to the brownie.
- Water helps to bring the batter together and create a smooth consistency.
- **Method:**

1. Mix dry ingredients in a mug: Start by adding the flour, sugar, and cocoa powder to a microwave-safe mug. Use a fork or small whisk to thoroughly mix the dry ingredients together until they are well combined and no lumps remain.

2. Add oil and water. Pour the oil and water into the mug with the dry ingredients. Use a fork or whisk to mix everything together until you have a smooth batter. Make sure to scrape down the sides and bottom of the mug to incorporate all the ingredients.

3. Microwave for 1-2 minutes until set. Place the mug in the microwave and cook on high power for 1-2 minutes. Cooking time may vary depending on the wattage of your microwave and the desired consistency of the brownie. Start with 1 minute, then check the brownie for doneness. It should be set around the edges but slightly gooey in the center. If it's still too wet, continue microwaving in 15–30 second intervals until cooked to your liking.

4. Let it cool: Once the brownie is cooked to your desired consistency, carefully remove the mug from the microwave using oven mitts, as it will be hot. Allow the brownie to cool for a few minutes before enjoying it directly from the mug or transferring it to a plate.

5. Optional toppings: You can enjoy the microwave mug brownie as is, or you can add toppings such as whipped cream, ice cream, chocolate sauce, or chopped nuts for extra flavor and texture.

Microwave mug brownies are a quick and easy dessert option when you're craving something sweet but don't want to go through the hassle of baking a full batch of brownies. Experiment with different add-ins like chocolate chips, nuts, or even a scoop of peanut butter to customize your brownie to your liking.

CHAPTER 7

Microwave Fish Fillets

Ingredients: fish fillets, lemon juice, salt, and pepper

1) **Method:** Season fish with lemon juice, salt, and pepper. Microwave on high for 3–4 minutes until cooked through. Ingredients:

2) Fish fillets: Choose your favorite type of fish fillet, such as tilapia, salmon, cod, or trout.

3) Lemon juice: Lemon juice adds flavor to the fish and helps to keep it moist during cooking.

4) Salt and pepper: Season the fish with salt and pepper to taste.

Method:

1. Prepare the fish fillets: Rinse the fish fillets under cold water and pat them dry with paper towels. Place the fillets on a microwave-safe plate or dish.

2. Season with lemon juice, salt, and pepper. Drizzle lemon juice over the fish fillets, ensuring they are evenly coated. Sprinkle salt and pepper over the fillets according to your taste preferences.

3. Microwave on high: Place the seasoned fish fillets in the microwave and cook on high power for 3–4 minutes. Cooking time may vary depending on the thickness and type of fish fillets you're using, as well as the power of your microwave. Start with 3 minutes, then check the fish for doneness. It should be opaque and flake easily with a fork when cooked through. If the fish is not fully cooked, continue microwaving in 30-second intervals until done.

4. Let it rest. Once the fish is cooked through, carefully remove it from the microwave using oven mitts, as the plate may be hot. Allow the fish to rest for a minute or two before serving. This allows the juices to redistribute and the fish to firm up slightly.

5. Serve: Transfer the cooked fish fillets to serving plates and garnish with additional lemon wedges, if desired. Serve immediately with your favorite side dishes, such as steamed vegetables, rice, or a fresh salad.

Microwaving fish fillets is a quick and convenient cooking method that yields tender and flavorful results. Experiment with different seasonings and marinades to customize the flavor of the fish to your liking. Enjoy this simple and healthy dish as a light lunch or dinner option.

CHAPTER 8

Microwave Rice

- o **Ingredients**: rice, water, and salt

Method: Rinse rice, add water, and salt in a microwave-safe dish. Microwave for 10–15 minutes, stirring halfway, until the rice is cooked. Certainly! Here's a more detailed explanation of how to cook rice in the microwave:

- **Ingredients:**
- Rice: Use your preferred type of rice, such as long-grain white rice, basmati rice, jasmine rice, brown rice, or any other variety.
- Water: The amount of water needed depends on the type of rice you're using and your preferred rice-to-water ratio. A general guideline is to use a ratio of 1 part rice to 2 parts water for white rice and 1 part rice to 2.5–3 parts water for brown rice.
- Salt: Salt is optional but can enhance the flavor of the rice.
- **Method:**

1. Rinse the rice: Place the rice in a fine-mesh strainer or sieve and rinse it under cold running water until the water runs clear. Rinsing helps to remove excess starch from the rice, resulting in fluffier cooked rice.

2. Add rice, water, and salt to a microwave-safe dish: Transfer the rinsed rice to a microwave-safe dish. Add the appropriate amount of water according to the type of rice you're using and your preferred rice-to-water ratio. If desired, add a pinch of salt for seasoning.

3. Cover the dish: Use a microwave-safe lid or microwave-safe plastic wrap to cover the dish. This helps to trap steam inside, which will cook the rice more evenly.

4. Microwave on high: Place the covered dish of rice and water in the microwave and cook on high power for 10–15 minutes, depending on the type of rice and the power of your microwave. Start with 10 minutes for white rice and 15 minutes for brown rice.

5. Stir halfway through cooking: About halfway through the cooking time, carefully remove the dish from the microwave and stir the rice with a fork to ensure even cooking and prevent sticking. If necessary, add a little more water if the rice seems too dry.

6. Continue cooking: Return the covered dish to the microwave and continue cooking until the rice is tender and all the water is absorbed. Check the rice for doneness by tasting a few grains. If it's still too firm, continue microwaving in 1-2 minute increments until cooked to your liking.

7. Let it rest. Once the rice is cooked, remove it from the microwave and let it rest, covered, for a few minutes.

8. This allows the rice to steam and finish cooking off the heat.

9. Fluff and serve: After resting, use a fork to fluff the rice, separating the grains. Serve the cooked rice as a side dish or as a base for your favorite rice-based recipes.

Microwaving rice is a quick and convenient method that yields fluffy and perfectly cooked rice. Experiment with different types of rice and seasoning variations to customize the flavor to your liking. Enjoy!

CHAPTER 9

Microwave-poached eggs

o **Ingredients:** eggs, water, vinegar, salt

Method: Fill a microwave-safe bowl with water and vinegar. Crack eggs into the water, cover with a plate, and microwave for 1-2 minutes until the whites are set. Here's a more detailed explanation of how to make microwave poached eggs:

- **Ingredients:**

Eggs: Use fresh eggs for best results.

- Water: sufficient water to fill the microwave-safe bowl.
- Vinegar: White vinegar or any other vinegar can be used. It helps the egg whites to set quickly.
- Salt: Optional for seasoning.
- **Method:**

1. Prepare the water. Fill a microwave-safe bowl with water, leaving enough space to submerge the eggs

completely. Add a splash of vinegar to the water. The vinegar helps the egg whites to coagulate faster resulting in a neater poached egg. You can also add a pinch of salt to the water for seasoning, if desired.

2. Microwave the water: Place the bowl of water in the microwave and heat it on high power for about 1-2 minutes, or until the water reaches a gentle simmer. Heating the water before adding the eggs helps to ensure that the eggs cook evenly.

3. Crack the eggs: Carefully crack the eggs, one at a time, into a small cup or ramekin. This makes it easier to slide the eggs into the hot water without breaking the yolks.

4. Add the eggs to the water. Once the water is simmering, gently slide the cracked eggs into the hot water, one at a time. Make sure to space them out evenly in the bowl. The eggs should be fully submerged in the water.

5. Microwave the eggs. Cover the bowl with a microwave-safe plate or lid to trap the steam and heat. Microwave the eggs on high power for 1-2 minutes, depending on your desired level of doneness. Cooking time may vary depending on the wattage of your microwave and how firm you like

6. your poached eggs. Check the eggs after 1 minute to see if the whites are set and the yolks are still runny. If not, continue microwaving in 15–30 second increments until done.

7. Remove and serve: Carefully remove the bowl from the microwave using oven mitts, as it will be hot. Use a slotted spoon to lift the poached eggs out of the water, allowing any excess water to drain off. Serve the poached eggs immediately while they're still warm, either on their own or atop toast, English muffins, or salads.

Microwave poached eggs are a quick and easy breakfast option that requires minimal effort and cleanup. Experiment with different cooking times to achieve your preferred level of doneness, whether you like your eggs soft and runny or more firm. Enjoy your perfectly poached eggs! Top of Form

CHAPTER 10

Microwave Bacon

o   Ingredients: Bacon slices

Method: Place bacon slices on a microwave-safe plate lined with paper towels. Microwave for 1-2 minutes per slice until crispy. Here's a more detailed explanation of how to microwave bacon:

- **Ingredients:**
- Bacon slices: Use your preferred type of bacon, such as regular, thick-cut, or turkey bacon.
- **Method:**

1. Prepare the microwave-safe plate: Line a microwave-safe plate with several layers of paper towels. The paper towels will absorb the excess grease as the bacon cooks and help to prevent splattering.
2. Arrange the bacon slices: Place the bacon slices in a single layer on the paper towel-lined plate. Make sure to space them out evenly and avoid overlapping to ensure even cooking.

3. Microwave the bacon: Place the plate of bacon in the microwave and cook on high power for 1-2 minutes per slice. Cooking time may vary depending on the thickness of the bacon slices and the desired level of crispiness. Start with 1 minute per slice, then check the bacon for doneness. If it's not yet crispy enough, continue microwaving in 30-second increments until it reaches your desired level of crispiness.

4. Check for doneness: Carefully remove the plate from the microwave using oven mitts, as it may be hot. Check the bacon for doneness by gently pressing on it with a fork or tongs. It should be browned and crispy.

5. Drain and serve: Once the bacon is cooked to your liking, transfer it to a plate lined with fresh paper towels to drain off any excess grease. Allow the bacon to cool for a minute or two before serving.

Microwaving bacon is a quick and convenient cooking method that produces crispy and delicious bacon without the need for a stovetop or oven. It's perfect for making a quick breakfast or adding crispy bacon to sandwiches, salads, or other dishes. Experiment with different cooking times to achieve your preferred level of crispiness, and enjoy your microwave bacon!

CHATER 11

Microwave Garlic Butter Shrimp

- **Ingredients:** shrimp, butter, garlic, lemon juice, salt, and pepper.

Method: Melt butter with minced garlic in a microwave-safe dish. Add shrimp, lemon juice, salt, and pepper. Microwave for 2–3 minutes until the shrimp are pink and cooked through. Here's a more detailed explanation of how to make microwave garlic butter shrimp:

Ingredients:

- Shrimp: Use fresh or thawed shrimp, peeled and deveined.
- Butter: Unsalted or salted butter can be used.
- Garlic: Freshly minced garlic or garlic paste adds flavor to the dish.
- Lemon juice: Freshly squeezed lemon juice adds brightness to the shrimp.
- Salt and pepper: seasonings to taste.

Method:

1. Prepare the microwave-safe dish: Use a microwave-safe dish large enough to hold the shrimp in a single layer. This ensures even cooking. You can use a glass or ceramic dish.

2. Melt butter with minced garlic. Place the butter in the microwave-safe dish and add the minced garlic. Microwave on high for about 30 seconds to 1 minute, or until the butter is melted and the garlic is fragrant. Keep an eye on it to prevent the butter from boiling over.

3. Add shrimp, lemon juice, salt, and pepper. Once the butter is melted, add the shrimp to the dish. Pour the lemon juice over the shrimp, and season with salt and pepper to taste. Toss the shrimp gently to coat them evenly with the garlic butter mixture.

4. Microwave the shrimp: Place the dish of shrimp in the microwave and cook on high power for 2-3 minutes, or until the shrimp are pink and opaque. Cooking time may vary depending on the size and quantity of shrimp and the power of your microwave. Be careful not to overcook the shrimp, as they can become tough and rubbery.

5. Check for doneness: Carefully remove the dish from the microwave using oven mitts, as it may be hot. Use a fork or knife to check the largest shrimp for doneness. They should be pink and opaque throughout.

6. Serve: Once the shrimp are cooked through, they are ready to serve. You can enjoy them hot as a main dish or appetizer, or you can add them to salads, pasta, or rice dishes for added flavor and protein.

Microwaving garlic butter shrimp is a quick and convenient way to prepare a delicious seafood dish with minimal cleanup. Experiment with different seasonings and variations to customize the recipe to your taste preferences. Enjoy your flavorful and succulent microwave garlic butter shrimp! Top of Form

CHAPTER 12

Microwave Mug Pizza

- o **Ingredients:** English muffin, pizza sauce, cheese, pepperoni (optional)

Method: Split the muffin, spread sauce, and top with cheese and pepperoni. Microwave Here's a more detailed explanation of how to make microwave mug pizza:

- **Ingredients:**

1. English muffin: You can use a whole English muffin or split it in half for two servings.
2. Pizza sauce: Use your favorite store-bought pizza sauce or homemade marinara sauce.
3. Cheese: Shredded mozzarella cheese works best, but you can use any type of cheese you prefer.
4. Pepperoni (optional): Add pepperoni slices for a classic pizza topping, or omit for a vegetarian option.

- **Method:**

1. Split and toast the English muffin (optional): If you prefer a crispy crust, split the English muffin in half

and lightly toast it in a toaster or toaster oven. This step is optional but adds texture to the pizza.

2. Spread pizza sauce. Place the English muffin halves in separate microwave-safe mugs or on a microwave-safe plate. Spread a spoonful of pizza sauce over each muffin half, covering it evenly from edge to edge.

3. Add cheese and toppings: sprinkle shredded cheese over the sauce-covered muffin halves, ensuring each muffin half is generously covered with cheese. If desired, add pepperoni slices or any other toppings of your choice.

4. Microwave the mug pizza: Place the mugs or plates with the prepared pizza in the microwave. Microwave on high power for 1-2 minutes, or until the cheese is melted and bubbly. Cooking time may vary depending on the wattage of your microwave and the thickness of the cheese.

5. Check for doneness: Carefully remove the mug pizza from the microwave using oven mitts, as the mug may be hot. Check to make sure the cheese is melted and bubbly, and the English muffin is heated through.

6. Let it cool and serve. Allow the mug pizza to cool for a minute or two before serving, as it will be hot. Enjoy

your microwave mug pizza as a quick and easy snack or meal!

Microwave mug pizza is a fun and convenient way to satisfy your pizza cravings in just a few minutes. You can customize the toppings to suit your taste preferences, making it a versatile and adaptable recipe. Experiment with different sauces, cheeses, and toppings to create your own personalized microwave mug pizza.

Top and bottom of the form

CHAPTER 13

Microwave-steamed broccoli with cheese

- ○ **Ingredients:** broccoli florets, cheese, water, salt
- ○ **Method:** Place the broccoli in a microwave-safe dish with water and salt. Microwave for 2–3 minutes. Top with cheese and microwave for another 30 seconds until the cheese is melted.

Here's a more detailed explanation of how to make microwave steamed broccoli with cheese:

- **Ingredients:**
- Broccoli florets: Use fresh broccoli florets, rinsed and trimmed.
- Cheese: Use shredded cheese of your choice, such as cheddar, mozzarella, or a blend.
- Water: Use water to create steam for steaming the broccoli.
- Salt: Optional for seasoning.
- Method:

1. Prepare the broccoli: Rinse the broccoli florets under cold water and trim off any tough stems or leaves. Cut the broccoli into bite-sized florets for even cooking.

2. Place the broccoli in a microwave-safe dish. Transfer the prepared broccoli florets to a microwave-safe dish. Add a small amount of water to the dish, enough to create steam but not so much that the broccoli is submerged. Sprinkle a pinch of salt over the broccoli for seasoning, if desired.

3. Microwave the broccoli: Cover the dish with a microwave-safe lid or microwave-safe plastic wrap to trap the steam inside. Microwave on high power for 2-3 minutes, or until the broccoli is tender-crisp. Cooking time may vary depending on the wattage of your microwave and the thickness of the broccoli florets.

4. Add cheese. Once the broccoli is steamed to your liking, remove the dish from the microwave. Sprinkle shredded cheese over the hot broccoli florets, covering them evenly with cheese.

5. Microwave to melt the cheese: Return the dish of broccoli to the microwave and microwave on high power for another 30 seconds, or until the cheese is

melted and bubbly. Keep an eye on it to prevent overcooking.

6. Serve: Carefully remove the dish from the microwave using oven mitts, as it may be hot. Serve the microwave steamed broccoli with cheese immediately as a side dish or as a topping for baked potatoes, rice, or pasta.

Microwave steamed broccoli with cheese is a quick and easy side dish that adds color, flavor, and nutrients to any meal. Experiment with different cheeses and seasoning variations to customize the dish to your taste preferences. Enjoy your delicious and nutritious microwave steamed broccoli with cheese!

CHAPTER 14

Microwave Nachos

- Ingredients: tortilla chips, cheese, salsa, and sour cream (optional).

Method: Arrange chips on a microwave-safe plate. Top it with cheese and salsa. Microwave for 1-2 minutes until the cheese is melted. Serve with sour cream, if desired. Here's a more detailed explanation of how to make microwave nachos:

• **Ingredients:**

- Tortilla chips: Use your favorite type of tortilla chips, such as corn or flavored varieties.
- Cheese: Shredded cheese works best for melting evenly. Cheddar, Monterey Jack, or a blend of cheeses are popular choices.
- Salsa: Choose your preferred salsa, whether it's mild, medium, or hot, depending on your taste preferences.
- Sour cream (optional): Sour cream adds creaminess and a cool contrast to the spicy flavors of the nachos.

- **Method:**

1. Arrange tortilla chips on a microwave-safe plate: Spread a single layer of tortilla chips evenly on a microwave-safe plate. Make sure to cover the entire surface of the plate without overlapping the chips.

2. Top with cheese: Sprinkle shredded cheese evenly over the tortilla chips, covering them generously with cheese. Use as much cheese as you like, depending on how cheesy you want your nachos to be.

3. Add salsa: Spoon salsa over the cheese-covered tortilla chips, distributing it evenly across the surface. You can use as much or as little salsa as you prefer, depending on how saucy you like your nachos.

4. Microwave the nachos: Place the plate of nachos in the microwave and cook on high power for 1-2 minutes, or until the cheese is melted and bubbly. Cooking time may vary depending on the wattage of your microwave and the amount of cheese you use. Keep an eye on the nachos to prevent them from burning.

5. Serve with sour cream (optional): Once the cheese is melted and bubbly, carefully remove the plate of nachos from the microwave using oven mitts, as it

may be hot. If desired, serve the nachos with a dollop of sour cream on the side for dipping.

6. Enjoy: Serve the microwave nachos immediately while they're still hot and crispy. Enjoy them as a delicious snack or appetizer, perfect for sharing with friends and family.

Microwave nachos are a quick and easy snack or appetizer that's perfect for movie nights, game days, or any casual gathering. Customize your nachos with additional toppings such as sliced jalapeños, black beans, diced tomatoes, or avocado slices to create your own signature nacho masterpiece.

CHAPTER 15

Microwave Mug Pancake

- o **Ingredients:** flour, milk, eggs, sugar, baking powder, and butter.
- o Method: Mix ingredients in a mug and microwave for 1-2 minutes until cooked through. Serve with syrup.

Here's a more detailed explanation of how to make microwave mug pancakes:

- **Ingredients:**
- Flour: Use all-purpose flour for this recipe.
- Milk: Any type of milk, such as cow's milk or plant-based milk, will work.
- Egg: Use a large egg.
- Sugar: Granulated sugar adds sweetness to the pancake batter.
- Baking powder: Baking powder helps the pancake rise and become fluffy.
- Butter: Melted butter adds richness to the pancake batter.
- **Method:**

1. Mix ingredients in a mug: In a microwave-safe mug, combine the flour, milk, egg, sugar, baking powder, and melted butter. Stir the ingredients together with a fork or small whisk until they are well combined and form a smooth batter. Make sure there are no lumps in the batter.

2. Microwave the mug pancake: Place the mug in the microwave and cook the pancake on high power for 1-2 minutes. Cooking time may vary depending on the wattage of your microwave and the size of your mug. Start with 1 minute and check for doneness. The pancake should be puffed up and set in the center.

3. Check for doneness: Carefully remove the mug from the microwave using oven mitts, as it may be hot. Insert a toothpick or fork into the center of the pancake to check if it's cooked through. If the toothpick comes out clean and the pancake is firm to the touch, it's done. If not, microwave for an additional 15–30 seconds until cooked through.

4. Serve with syrup: Once the pancake is cooked through, drizzle it with your favorite syrup or toppings. Maple syrup, honey, fruit compote, or chocolate sauce are all delicious options. Enjoy your

microwave mug pancake immediately while it's still warm.

Microwave mug pancakes are a quick and convenient breakfast option for busy mornings or when you're craving a homemade pancake but don't want to make a whole batch. Customize your pancake by adding chocolate chips, blueberries, or sliced bananas to the batter before microwaving for extra flavor and texture.

CHAPTER 16

Microwave-stuffed bell peppers

- **Ingredients**: bell peppers, ground beef or turkey, rice, tomato sauce, cheese, salt, and pepper
- Method: Cut the tops off peppers, remove the seeds. Mix cooked ground meat, cooked rice, tomato sauce, cheese, salt, and pepper. Stuff peppers and microwave for 5-7 minutes until they are tender.

Here's a more detailed explanation of how to make microwave stuffed bell peppers:

- **Ingredients:**
- Bell peppers: Choose bell peppers of any color you prefer, such as red, yellow, or green.
- Ground beef or turkey: Use cooked ground meat for the filling. You can use beef, turkey, or any other ground meat of your choice.
- Rice: Use cooked rice as part of the filling. White rice, brown rice, or any other type of rice will work.
- Tomato sauce: Tomato sauce adds flavor and moisture to the filling. You can use store-bought tomato sauce or homemade marinara sauce.

- Cheese: Shredded cheese adds richness and flavor to the filling. Cheddar, mozzarella, or a blend of cheeses work well.

- Salt and pepper: seasonings to taste.

- **Method:**

1. Prepare the bell peppers: Cut the tops off the bell peppers and remove the seeds and membranes from the inside. Rinse the peppers under cold water to remove any remaining seeds.

2. Prepare the filling: In a mixing bowl, combine the cooked ground meat, cooked rice, tomato sauce, shredded cheese, salt, and pepper. Stir the ingredients together until they are well combined and form a cohesive mixture.

3. Stuff the peppers: Spoon the filling mixture into the hollowed-out bell peppers, packing it down firmly to fill the peppers completely. You can mound the filling slightly on top if needed.

4. Microwave the stuffed peppers: Place the stuffed peppers in a microwave-safe dish, arranging them so they are standing upright. Cover the dish with a microwave-safe lid or microwave-safe plastic wrap to trap steam inside. Microwave the stuffed peppers on high power for 5-7 minutes, or until the peppers are

tender and the filling is heated through. Cooking time may vary depending on the size and thickness of the peppers.

5. Check for doneness: Carefully remove the dish from the microwave using oven mitts, as it may be hot. Use a fork or knife to test the tenderness of the peppers. They should be easily pierced with a fork or knife, indicating that they are cooked through.

6. Serve: Once the stuffed peppers are cooked through, carefully remove them from the microwave and serve them immediately. You can enjoy them as a satisfying main dish or as part of a meal with a side salad or steamed vegetables.

Microwave stuffed bell peppers are a convenient and flavorful dish that's perfect for a quick and easy weeknight dinner. Customize the filling with your favorite ingredients, such as diced vegetables, beans, or herbs, to suit your taste preferences. Enjoy your delicious microwave stuffed bell peppers. Top of Form

CHAPTER 17

Microwave-mashed potatoes

- Ingredients: potatoes, butter, milk, salt, and pepper
- Method: Peel and chop potatoes; place in a microwave-safe dish with water. Microwave for 8–10 minutes until tender. Mash with butter, milk, salt, and pepper.
- Here's a more detailed explanation of how to make microwave mashed potatoes:
- **Ingredients:**
- Potatoes: Use your preferred type of potatoes, such as russet potatoes or Yukon Gold potatoes.
- Butter: Unsalted or salted butter adds richness and flavor to the mashed potatoes.
- Milk: Any type of milk, such as whole milk, low-fat milk, or plant-based milk, can be used to adjust the consistency of the mashed potatoes.
- Salt and pepper: seasonings to taste.
- **Method:**

1. Prepare the potatoes: Peel the potatoes and cut them into evenly sized chunks to ensure even cooking.

Rinse the potato chunks under cold water to remove any excess starch.

2. Microwave the potatoes: Place the potato chunks in a microwave-safe dish and add enough water to cover them completely. Microwave the potatoes on high power for 8–10 minutes, or until they are tender when pierced with a fork. Cooking time may vary depending on the size and type of potatoes, as well as the wattage of your microwave.

3. Drain the potatoes. Carefully remove the dish from the microwave using oven mitts, as it may be hot. Use a colander to drain the water from the cooked potatoes.

4. Mash the potatoes. Transfer the drained potatoes to a mixing bowl. Add butter, milk, salt, and pepper to the bowl. Use a potato masher or fork to mash the potatoes until they reach your desired level of smoothness. For creamier mashed potatoes, you can use an electric hand mixer or potato ricer.

5. Adjust seasoning and consistency: Taste the mashed potatoes and adjust the seasoning with additional salt and pepper, if needed. If the mashed potatoes are too thick, you can add more milk to achieve the desired consistency.

6. Serve: Once the mashed potatoes are seasoned to your liking and have reached the desired consistency, they are ready to serve. Transfer the mashed potatoes to a serving dish and garnish with a pat of butter or a sprinkle of chopped parsley, if desired. Serve the mashed potatoes hot as a side dish with your favorite main course.

Microwave mashed potatoes are a quick and easy side dish that pairs well with a variety of meals. Experiment with different variations, such as adding roasted garlic, sour cream, or herbs, to customize the flavor of your mashed potatoes. Enjoy your creamy and delicious microwave mashed potatoes. Top of Form

CHAPTER 18

Microwave Mug Lasagna

Ingredients: lasagna noodles, ricotta cheese, marinara sauce, mozzarella cheese, salt, and pepper.

Method: Break noodles into a mug and layer with ricotta, sauce, and mozzarella. Microwave for 2–3 minutes until the cheese is melted. Here's a more detailed explanation of how to make microwave mug lasagna:

- **Ingredients:**
- Lasagna noodles: Use dried lasagna noodles, broken into pieces to fit the mug.
- Ricotta cheese: Creamy ricotta cheese adds richness and flavor to the lasagna.
- Marinara sauce: Use your favorite marinara sauce, either store-bought or homemade.
- Mozzarella cheese: Shredded mozzarella cheese adds gooey, cheesy goodness to the lasagna.
- Salt and pepper: seasonings to taste.
- **Method:**

1. Prepare the lasagna noodles: Break the lasagna noodles into small pieces that will fit comfortably into the mug. You can break them by hand or use a knife to cut them into smaller pieces.

2. Layer the lasagna in the mug: Start by placing a layer of lasagna noodles in the bottom of the mug. Add a spoonful of ricotta cheese on top of the noodles, spreading it evenly to cover the noodles. Next, spoon marinara sauce over the ricotta cheese layer, followed by a sprinkle of shredded mozzarella cheese. Repeat the layer until the mug is filled, finishing with a layer of mozzarella cheese on top.

3. Microwave the mug lasagna: Place the mug in the microwave and microwave on high power for 2-3 minutes, or until the cheese is melted and bubbly. Cooking time may vary depending on the wattage of your microwave and the size of your mug. Keep an eye on the lasagna to prevent it from bubbling over.

4. Check for doneness: Carefully remove the mug from the microwave using oven mitts, as it may be hot. Use a fork or knife to test the tenderness of the noodles and ensure they are cooked through. The cheese should be melted and bubbly, and the sauce should be hot.

5. Let it cool and serve: Allow the mug lasagna to cool for a minute or two before serving, as it will be very hot. Enjoy your microwave mug lasagna straight from the mug, or carefully transfer it to a plate or bowl for easier eating.

1. Microwave mug lasagna is a quick and easy meal that's perfect for a satisfying lunch or dinner. Customize your mug lasagna with additional ingredients, such as cooked ground meat, sautéed vegetables, or fresh herbs, to suit your taste preferences. Enjoy your delicious and convenient microwave mug lasagna!

CHAPTER 19

Microwave Sweet Potatoes

Ingredients: Graham crackers, chocolate, marshmallows

Method: Assemble crackers, chocolate, and marshmallows. Microwave for 10–20 seconds until marshmallows puff and chocolate melts.

Here's a more detailed explanation of how to make microwave sweet potatoes, certainly! Here's a detailed explanation of how to make microwave sweet potatoes:

- **Ingredients:**
- Sweet potatoes: Choose medium-sized sweet potatoes that are firm and without blemishes. Wash and scrub them thoroughly before cooking.
- **Method:**

1. Prepare the sweet potatoes: Use a fork to pierce the sweet potatoes several times on all sides. This allows steam to escape during cooking and prevents the sweet potatoes from bursting in the microwave.
2. Microwave the sweet potatoes. Place the prepared sweet potatoes on a microwave-safe plate or dish.

Microwave them on high power for 5-7 minutes per potato, depending on the size and wattage of your microwave. Turn the sweet potatoes over halfway through the cooking time to ensure even cooking.

3. Check for doneness: Carefully remove the plate from the microwave using oven mitts, as it may be hot. Use a fork or knife to test the tenderness of the sweet potatoes. They should be soft and easily pierced with a fork when they are done. If the sweet potatoes are not cooked through, continue microwaving them in 1-2 minute increments until they reach the desired level of tenderness.

4. Let them rest. Once the sweet potatoes are cooked through, allow them to rest for a few minutes before handling. This allows the steam to escape and the sweet potatoes to cool slightly.

5. Serve and enjoy. Slice open the cooked sweet potatoes and serve them hot. You can enjoy them plain or with your favorite toppings, such as butter, cinnamon, brown sugar, marshmallows, or chopped nuts.

Microwaving sweet potatoes is a quick and convenient way to cook them, especially when you're short on time. They make a delicious and nutritious side dish or can be enjoyed as a satisfying main course when topped with your favorite ingredients. Experiment with different toppings and seasonings to create your own unique microwave sweet potato recipe.

CHAPTER 20

Microwave Garlic Bread

- **Ingredients**: bread slices, butter, garlic powder, parsley

Method: Spread butter on bread and sprinkle with garlic powder and parsley. Microwave for 30–60 seconds until the butter melts and the bread is toasted. Here's a more detailed explanation of how to make microwave garlic bread:

- **Ingredients:**
- Bread slices: Use your preferred type of bread, such as white bread, whole wheat bread, or French bread.
- Butter: Use softened butter or margarine for spreading on the bread.
- Garlic powder: Garlic powder adds flavor to the garlic bread.
- Parsley: Chopped parsley adds color and freshness to the garlic bread (optional).
- **Method:**

1. Prepare the bread. Position the slices of bread on a microwave-safe dish or plate. Make sure they are

stacked without overlapping on top of each other. Spread butter on the bread: Using a knife or butter spreader evenly spread softened butter or margarine on one side of each slice of bread. Make sure the butter is all over the edges of the bread. Parsley and garlic powder for sprinkling: Make sure to evenly coat the entire surface of each slice of bread with garlic powder on the buttered side. If desired, sprinkle chopped parsley on top of the garlic powder for added flavor and aesthetic appeal. Place the bread with garlic in the microwave. Place the bread plate with sautéed garlic on it. in the microwave. 30–60 minutes at high power in the microwave, or until the butter melts and the bread is toasted to your liking. Cooking time may vary depending on the wattage of your microwave and the thickness of the bread slices. Keep an eye on the garlic bread to prevent it from burning.

2. Check for doneness: Carefully remove the plate from the microwave using oven mitts, as it may be hot. Check the garlic bread to ensure that the butter is melted and the bread is toasted to your desired level of crispiness.

3. Serve and enjoy: Once the garlic bread is cooked to your liking, remove it from the microwave and serve it

immediately. Enjoy the warm and flavorful garlic bread as a delicious side dish or appetizer with your favorite meals.

Microwave garlic bread is a quick and convenient way to enjoy the delicious flavors of garlic and butter without the need for an oven. Experiment with different types of bread and additional seasonings to customize the garlic bread to your taste preferences. Enjoy your homemade microwave garlic bread as a tasty accompaniment to any meal!

These recipes provide a variety of easy-to-make meals and snacks using the microwave, perfect for beginners looking for quick and delicious options.

CHAPTER 21

Breakfast burrito in a mug:

This recipe calls for eggs, cheese, and vegetables including sp inach and bell peppers.

It's a quick and easy breakfast choice that's high in protein a nd vital nutrients

Here is a microwave breakfast burrito recipe in a mug, along with a list of its nutritional advantages:

Ingredients include one large egg, two tablespoons each of m ilk and shredded cheese, one tablespoon each of salsa, and o ne small flour tortilla. - Season with salt and pepper.

Guidelines:

1. Crack the egg and pour the milk into a mug that is safe to microwave.

Using a fork, beat together until thoroughly mixed.

2. Add the salsa, salt, pepper, and shredded cheese and stir.

3. Break up the flour tortilla into little pieces and mix them t horoughly with the egg mixture to coat them.

4. Cook the egg in the mug in the microwave for one to two minutes on high, stirring halfway through.

5. The mug will be hot, so take care while taking it out of the microwave and

Nutritional Advantages:

Eggs are a great source of complete protein since they contain every necessary amino acid.
They also include choline, which is necessary for the growth and health of the brain. - Milk provides

CHAPTER 22

Microwave Mug Quiche

2.   A tasty and filling dish composed of eggs, milk, cheese, a nd cooked meat or a variety of vegetables.

It's a fantastic source of protein and may be tailored to contain the ingredients of your   choice. Certainly! Here's a recipe for Microwave Mug Quiche, along with its method and nutritional benefits, particularly for diabetes patients:

Ingredients:

- 1 large egg

- 2 tablespoons milk (low-fat or skim)

- 2 tablespoons chopped vegetables (such as spinach, bell peppers, or mushrooms)

- 1 tablespoon shredded cheese (low-fat or reduced-fat)

- Salt and pepper, to taste

Instructions:

1. In a microwave-safe mug, crack the egg and add the milk. Beat together with a fork until well combined.

2. Stir in the chopped vegetables, shredded cheese, salt,

and pepper.

3. Microwave the mug on high for about 1 minute. Check the consistency of the quiche - if it needs more time to cook through, microwave in additional 15-second intervals until set.

4. Carefully remove the mug from the microwave (it will be hot) and let it cool for a minute before enjoying your Microwave Mug Quiche.

Nutritional Benefits:

For diabetes patients specifically:

- One large egg provides about 6 grams of high-quality protein while being low in carbohydrates.

- Low-fat or skim milk adds calcium and vitamin D without adding excessive fat or sugar.

- Vegetables like spinach, bell peppers, or mushrooms are low in carbohydrates but rich in fiber and essential nutrients like vitamins A and C.

- Shredded cheese can add flavor without adding too much saturated fat if you choose a low-fat or reduced-fat variety.

Overall, this Microwave Mug Quiche provides balanced nutrients with protein from eggs and dairy products while being lower in carbohydrates due to minimal crust-like ingredients commonly found in traditional quiches. The addition of vegetables adds essential fiber that can help regulate blood sugar levels for diabetes patients.

CHAPTER 23

Microwave Mug Chili:

Certainly! Here's a recipe for Microwave Mug Chili along with the detailed preparation of ingredients and nutritional benefits:

Ingredients:
- 1/4 cup lean ground turkey or beef (cooked)
- 2 tablespoons diced onion
- 2 tablespoons diced bell pepper
- 2 tablespoons canned kidney beans (rinsed and drained)
- 2 tablespoons canned diced tomatoes
- 1/4 teaspoon chili powder
- 1/8 teaspoon cumin
- Salt and pepper to taste

Method:

1. In a microwave-safe mug, combine the cooked ground turkey or beef, diced onion, diced bell pepper, kidney beans, diced tomatoes, chili powder, cumin, salt, and

pepper.

2. Stir well to combine all the ingredients.

3. Cover the mug loosely with a microwave-safe plate or microwave-safe plastic wrap.

4. Microwave on high for about 2 minutes.

5. Carefully remove from the microwave (mug will be hot) and stir well.

6. Return to the microwave and cook for an additional minute or until heated through.

Nutritional Benefits for Diabetes Patients:

Lean Ground Turkey or Beef: Lean protein sources like turkey or beef provide essential amino acids without significantly affecting blood sugar levels.

Onion: Onions are low in carbohydrates and calories but rich in flavor and nutrients like vitamin C and dietary fiber that aid in blood sugar control.

Bell Pepper: Bell peppers add crunchiness to the dish while providing an excellent source of vitamin C,vitamin A,and dietary fibers that help maintain stable blood sugar levels.

Kidney Beans: Kidney beans are a good source of plant-based protein, fiber, and essential minerals like magnesium which helps control blood sugar levels. They also have a low glycolic index value that minimizes spikes in blood glucose after consumption.

Diced Tomatoes: Diced tomatoes are low in calories but packed with beneficial nutrients like vitamins A,C,and lycopene—an antioxidant known to have potential health benefits including reducing inflammation.

Chili Powder & Cumin: Both spices add flavor without adding excessive sodium, sugar, fat, or carbohydrates which can negatively affect blood sugar control.

Overall,this Microwave Mug Chili recipe provides lean proteins from ground turkey/beef, fiber from onions, bell peppers, kidney beans, diced tomatoes, and beneficial spices with low glycolic index values. These ingredients together help maintain stable blood sugar levels while providing essential nutrients necessary for overall health management in diabetes patients

CHAPTER 24

Macaroni and cheese in a microwave Mug with broccoli

 Calcium from cheese helps build healthy bones. Br rtainly! Here's a recipe for Macaroni and Cheese in a Microwave Mug with Broccoli along with the detailed preparation of ingredients and nutritional benefits:

Ingredients:

- 1/3 cup elbow macaroni
- 1/2 cup water
- 1/4 cup milk (low-fat or skim)
- 1/2 cup shredded cheddar cheese (low-fat or reduced-fat)
- 1/4 cup chopped broccoli florets
- Salt and pepper to taste

Method:

1. In a microwave-safe mug, combine the elbow macaroni and water.

2. Microwave on high for about 2 minutes, stirring

halfway through, until the macaroni is cooked.

3. Drain any excess water from the mug.

4. Add the milk, shredded cheddar cheese, chopped broccoli florets, salt, and pepper to the mug with the cooked macaroni.

5. Stir well to combine all the ingredients.

6. Microwave on high for another minute or until the cheese is melted and bubbly.

7. Carefully remove from the microwave (mug will be hot) and let it cool slightly before serving.

Nutritional Benefits for Diabetes Patients:

Elbow Macaroni: Whole grain options of elbow macaroni provide dietary fiber that slows down digestion and helps regulate blood sugar levels.

Milk: Low-fat or skim milk is a good source of calcium, vitamin D, and protein. Choosing low-fat options helps manage weight while providing essential nutrients without excessive saturated fat.

Shredded Cheddar Cheese: Opting for low-fat or reduced-fat shredded cheddar cheese provides flavor without adding excessive saturated fat. It also contains protein as well as essential vitamins like vitamin B12 which is important for nerve function.

Broccoli: Broccoli provides dietary fiber,vitamin C,vitamin K,and folate which are beneficial nutrients associated with blood sugar control.Choosing vegetables like broccoli adds bulk to meals without significantly increasing calorie intake.They also have a low glycemic index value that minimizes spikes in blood glucose after consumption.

Overall, this Macaroni and Cheese in a Microwave Mug with Broccoli recipe incorporates whole grain pasta, dairy protein,and nutrient-dense broccoli resulting in a balanced meal option.While providing essential nutrients,it also helps maintain stable blood sugar levels due to its lower glycemic index values
occoli is high in dietary fiber, folate, vitamins C and K, and fo late. 5.

CHAPTER 25

Egg Fried Rice in a Microwave Mug

Numerous essential elements, including as vitamins A, B12, D, E, and K; riboflavin; protein; selenium; choline; lutein; and zeaxanthin, are abundant in eggs.

A rich source of vitamins A, C, K, E, choline, and folic acid, spinach also contains significant amounts of magnesium, p

Of course!

Here's a recipe for Microwave Mug Eggs Fried Rice, complete with instructions and nutritional value—

especially for those with diabetes—for this dish:

Components: -

Half a cup of cooked rice, ideally brown rice for extra fiber -

One egg -

Two teaspoons of mixed veggies, like bell peppers, carrots, and peas - A tablespoon of soy sauce with reduced sodium -

As an optional garnish, you can add soons or sesame seeds.

Instructions:

1. Place the mixed vegetables and cooked rice in a microwave-safe mug.

2. Crack the egg right into the mug containing the veggies and rice. 3. Pour the low-

sodium soy sauce over the mug's contents.

4. Gently whisk the egg with a fork and stir all the ingredient s together until thoroughly blended.

5. after about a minute on high, turn the microwave ofotassiu m, and iron. 8.

CHAPTER 26

Microwave Artichoke Dip with Spinach

The nutritional profile of spinach is remarkable, containing d
ietary fibers, magnesium, zinc, folic acid, vitamin K, and vita
mins A, C, and E. -

Research has demonstrated that asparagus promotes heart h
ealth, liver function, and digestion.They're also a fantastic so
urce of magnesium, potassium, and the vitamins C, K, E, and
 B6.

Depending on the components used, these dishes can offer a
balance of essential micronutrients (vitamins and minerals) t
ogether with macronutrients (carbohydrates, protein, and fac
t)To optimize nutritional advantages, it's a good idea to use
whole food products whenever possible! .

Naturally, of course! Here are a few additional mic on how to
prepare it

Ingredients:

- 1 cup chopped spinach (fresh or frozen)
- 1 can (14 oz) artichoke hearts, drained and chopped
- 1 cup shredded mozzarella cheese
- 1/2 cup grated Parmesan cheese

- 1/2 cup mayonnaise or Greek yogurt
- 1/4 cup sour cream
- 2 cloves garlic, minced
- Salt and pepper to taste

Instructions:

1. In a microwave-safe dish, mix together the chopped spinach, chopped artichoke hearts, mozzarella cheese, Parmesan cheese, mayonnaise or Greek yogurt, sour cream, minced garlic, salt and pepper.
2. Microwave the mixture on high for about 3 minutes or until the cheeses are melted and the dip is heated through.
3. Stir the dip well to combine all ingredients evenly.
4. If needed, heat for an additional minute or until fully heated.

This warm and creamy Microwave Artichoke Dip with Spinach is perfect for serving at gatherings as a delicious appetizer!

As for nutritional benefits specifically related to diabetes patients:
- Spinach is low in carbohydrates and calories while being high in fiber which helps regulate blood sugar levels.

- Artichoke hearts are also low in carbohydrates and are a good source of fiber as well as vitamins C and K.
- Using Greek yogurt instead of mayonnaise can add protein without extra sugars typically found in some commercial mayonnaise products.

It's important for diabetes patients to be mindful of portion sizes due to potential high fat content from cheeses and mayonnaise/sour cream. It's always best to consult with a healthcare professional or registered dietitian when considering new recipes or ingredients.

CHAPTER 27

Microwave Mug Chicken Alfredo Pasta

Lean protein sources like chicken aid in tissue growth and re
pair. -

Pasta offers carbohydrates that are abundant in energy, and
sauce enhances flavor but should be consumed

 ingredients:

- 1/2 cup cooked pasta (such as fettuccine or penne)

- 1/4 cup cooked chicken breast, diced

- 1/4 cup frozen peas

- 1/4 cup grated Parmesan cheese

- 2 tablespoons unsalted butter or olive oil

- 2 tablespoons heavy cream or milk

- Salt and pepper to taste

Instructions:

1. In a microwave-safe mug, combine the cooked pasta, diced
chicken breast, frozen peas, grated Parmesan cheese, butter
or olive oil, heavy cream or milk.

2. Stir all the ingredients together until well combined.

3. Microwave on high for about 1 minute and stir gently.

4. Continue microwaving in 30-second intervals until the

sauce is heated through and the cheese is melted.

5. Season with salt and pepper to taste before enjoying your Microwave Mug Chicken Alfredo Pasta.

Nutritional Benefits:

Chicken Alfredo pasta can be a satisfying dish when prepared in a healthier way:

For protein:
- Chicken breast provides lean protein that can help build and repair tissues while assisting with blood sugar control.
For carbohydrates:
- Using whole wheat pasta instead of refined white pasta increases fiber content which promotes better blood sugar management by slowing down digestion.

For vegetables:
- The addition of frozen peas provides vitamins A, C, K as well as fiber while adding texture and color to the dish.
For fats:
- Using unsalted butter or olive oil helps control sodium intake while providing healthy fats that are beneficial for heart health.

Overall, this Microwave Mug Chicken Alfredo Pasta recipe offers balanced nutrients with lean protein from chicken breast along with wholesome carbohydrates from whole wheat pasta. It includes vegetables for added nutrients like fiber and vitamins while being mindful of fat content by using unsalted butter or olive oil in moderation.

It's important to note that portion sizes should be considered based on individual dietary needs and goals. Consulting with a healthcare professional or registered dietitian is recommended for personalized

guidance regarding nutritional needs associated with diabetes management

CHAPTER 28

Mexican Rice Bowl in Microwave Mug

Rice contains tiny amounts of protein and carbs for energy. Black beans include fiber, plant-b ingredients:

- 1/4 cup cooked brown rice
- 1/4 cup canned black beans, rinsed and drained
- 2 tablespoons salsa
- 2 tablespoons diced tomatoes
- 2 tablespoons diced red bell pepper
- 2 tablespoons grated cheddar cheese
- Optional toppings: chopped avocado, sour cream (use light or Greek yogurt alternative), chopped cilantro

Preparation:

1. In a microwave-safe mug, combine the cooked brown rice, black beans, salsa, diced tomatoes, and diced red bell pepper.

2. Stir the ingredients together until well mixed.

3. Microwave on high for about 1 minute and stir gently.

4. Continue microwaving in 30-second intervals until everything is heated through.

5. Sprinkle grated cheddar cheese on top and microwave for an additional 15-30 seconds until the cheese melts.

6. Add optional toppings such as chopped avocado, sour cream (or a light/Greek yogurt alternative), and chopped

cilantro before serving your Microwave Mexican Rice Bowl.

Nutritional Benefits for Diabetes Patients:

This recipe offers several nutritional benefits that can suit diabetes patients:

For carbohydrates:

- Brown rice is a whole grain that provides complex carbohydrates with fiber, which helps regulate blood sugar levels.

For protein and fiber:

- Black beans are an excellent source of plant-based protein while also being rich in dietary fiber to promote satiety and support steady blood sugar control.

For vegetables:

- Diced tomatoes and red bell peppers add essential vitamins such as vitamin C along with dietary fiber to aid digestion.

For fats:

- Grated cheddar cheese adds flavor while providing healthy fats in moderation.

Optional toppings considerations:

- Avocado is a good source of heart-friendly monounsaturated fats along with vitamins C, E, K, B6.

(Note: Diabetes patients should moderate their intake due to its high calorie content.)

Overall, this Microwave Mexican Rice Bowl recipe offers a balance of complex carbs from brown rice enhanced by dietary fiber-rich black beans. It incorporates various vegetables for added nutrients like vitamins C and A while using moderate amounts of healthy fats from cheese or avocado if included as toppings.

Always consult with a healthcare professional or registered dietitian for personalized advice on managing
diabetes through appropriate portion control tailored to individual needs.

CHAPTER 29

. Microwave Chicken Parmesan:

-Chicken provides lean proteins along with important nutrients such as niacin,Vitamin B6,Vitamin B12,Zinc,Selenium

Here's a recipe for Microwave Chicken Parmesan along with the ingredients, method, and nutritional benefits for diabetes patients:

Ingredients:

- 2 boneless, skinless chicken breasts
- 1/2 cup whole wheat bread crumbs
- 1/4 cup grated Parmesan cheese
- 1/4 teaspoon garlic powder
- 1/4 teaspoon dried oregano
- 1/4 teaspoon dried basil
- Salt and pepper to taste
- 1/2 cup marinara sauce (low sugar or homemade)
- 1/2 cup shredded mozzarella cheese

Method:

1. In a shallow bowl, mix together the bread crumbs, Parmesan cheese, garlic powder, dried oregano, dried basil, salt, and pepper.

2. Dip each chicken breast into the bread crumb mixture to coat both sides.

3. Place the coated chicken breasts on a microwave-safe plate or baking dish.

4. Microwave on high for about 5 minutes or until the chicken is cooked through.

5. Remove from the microwave and spoon marinara sauce over each chicken breast.

6. Sprinkle shredded mozzarella cheese over the top of each breast.

7. Microwave again on high for about 30 seconds or until the cheese is melted.

Nutritional Benefits for Diabetes Patients:

Chicken: Lean proteins like chicken are essential for maintaining stable blood sugar levels as they do not cause significant spikes in blood glucose levels. Additionally, chicken is rich in niacin (vitamin B3), vitamin B6, vitamin B12, zinc, and selenium which play important roles in maintaining overall health and supporting optimal metabolic function.

Whole Wheat Bread Crumbs: Using whole wheat bread crumbs instead of white bread crumbs adds more fiber to the dish which can help slow down digestion and reduce sudden increases in blood sugar levels.

Marinara Sauce: Opting for low-sugar marinara sauce or making your own allows you to control the amount of added sugars while still enjoying the flavors of tomatoes that are rich in vitamins A and C.

Parmesan Cheese: While it should be used in moderation due to its higher fat content, parmesan cheese adds a burst of flavor without adding excessive carbohydrates that can impact blood sugar levels.

Overall, this Microwave Chicken Parmesan recipe provides lean protein from chicken along with important nutrients like niacin (vitamin B3), vitamin B6,vitamin B12,zinc,selenium.This meal also incorporates whole grains from whole wheat breadcrumbs and beneficial vitamins from marinara sauce while keeping added sugars low.

CHAPTER 30

Microwave Mug Stuffed Bell Peppers

-Bell peppers provide an excellent source of vitamin Here's a recipe for Microwave Mug Stuffed Bell Peppers along with the method of preparation and nutritional benefits for diabetes patients:

Ingredients:

- 1 bell pepper (any color)
- 1/4 cup cooked quinoa
- 1/4 cup lean ground turkey or chicken (cooked)
- 2 tablespoons diced tomatoes
- 2 tablespoons grated low-fat cheese
- Salt and pepper to taste

Method:

1. Cut off the top of the bell pepper and remove the seeds and white membrane.

2. In a microwave-safe mug, mix together the cooked quinoa, ground turkey or chicken, diced tomatoes, grated cheese, salt, and pepper.

3. Spoon the mixture into the hollowed-out bell pepper.

4. Cover the mug loosely with a microwave-safe plate or microwave-safe plastic wrap.

5. Microwave on high for about 3-4 minutes or until the bell pepper is tender.

Nutritional Benefits for Diabetes Patients:

Bell Peppers: Bell peppers are low in carbohydrates and calories while being rich in vitamins C and A. Vitamin C helps in boosting immunity while vitamin A is important for maintaining healthy vision. Additionally, they provide dietary fiber that aids in blood sugar control by slowing down digestion.

Quinoa: Quinoa is a nutritious whole grain that contains protein, fiber, vitamins (B vitamins), minerals (such as magnesium), antioxidants, and phyto nutrients. It has a lower glycemic index than some other grains like rice or pasta which means it has less impact on blood sugar levels.

Lean Ground Turkey or Chicken: Lean protein sources like turkey or chicken are beneficial for diabetes patients as they provide essential amino acids without significantly affecting blood sugar levels.

Tomatoes: Tomatoes are low in calories but packed with

beneficial nutrients like vitamins A and C as well as lycopene—an antioxidant known to have potential health benefits including reducing inflammation.

Low-Fat Cheese: Using grated low-fat cheese adds flavor without adding excessive saturated fat or carbohydrates that can negatively affect blood sugar levels.

Overall, this Microwave Mug Stuffed Bell Peppers recipe provides an excellent source of vitamin C,vitamin A,and dietary fibers from bell peppers while incorporating nutrient-dense ingredients like quinoa,turkey/chicken,tomatoes,and low-fat cheese.All these ingredients help maintain stable blood sugar levels due to their lower glycemic index values while providing essential nutrients necessary for overall health management in diabetes patients

C,vitamin A,and dietary fibers

CONCLUSION

In conclusion, while microwave foods offer convenience and efficiency, their impact on nutrition remains a subject of scrutiny. Despite concerns regarding potential nutrient loss and alterations in food composition, technological advancements continue to improve microwave cooking methods, aiming to minimize nutritional compromise. However, consumers must remain vigilant and informed, understanding that not all microwave meals are created equal in terms of nutritional value. Balanced nutrition is paramount, and reliance solely on microwave foods may lead to deficiencies or imbalances in essential nutrients. Thus, it's crucial to complement microwave meals with fresh, whole foods whenever possible, ensuring a diverse and nutrient-rich diet. Moreover, prudent selection of microwave meals, focusing on options with minimal processing and additives, can mitigate potential health risks associated with heavily processed convenience foods. Ultimately, while microwave foods offer unparalleled convenience in today's fast-paced world, prioritizing   nutrition and mindful consumption is key to achieving optimal health and well-being.

Congratulation for chosen this book enjoy your kitchen